Being A Good Patient Can Save Your Life

A guide to improve your medical care
now and long term.

Alexander L Sytman M.D.

ISBN: 1484150422
ISBN 13: 9781484150429

Dedication

This book is dedicated to my wife and children, who encouraged me to help my patients by teaching them to better advocate for their own well-being. My life's work would not have been possible without their encouragement for so many years during my training and practice of internal medicine and cardiology. I also dedicate this book to my many medical colleagues, staff, technicians, and all the wonderful office and hospital nurses who made my life work such a joy.

My quest for patient advocacy was also inspired by all of the terrific office nurses who enhanced my out-of-hospital work from July 1970 to December 2010. Special thanks go to the last two registered nurses who helped me care for my dear patients over the span of several years at Minor & James Medical Clinic in Seattle before my retirement in 2010 — Christina Roeun and Diana Armstrong.

Contents

Introduction

When I was in medical school, one of my most interesting professors was an internal medicine doctor working in the department of psychiatry. His specialty was psychophysiology: the body's response to psychological stress. He believed that all diseases had an associated mental attitude or personality. His research led him to the conclusion that our attitudes can shape the way our bodies behave physically and chemically. "To be successfully sick, you have to start early in life," he once said.

One of my classmates encountered a patient who, when asked, "When did your illness begin?" responded, "Well, I was a breech delivery." I'm not certain if my classmate was joking or if his patient really said that. If the anecdote was true, this response suggests that our professor may well have been correct about what it takes to be successfully sick. But today I believe the opposite: to be successfully healthy, you have to start early in life. Good parents will foster this approach to health for their children, beginning before their children's birth by getting good prenatal care, but it's never too late to begin preventive care, even in later life. I firmly believe we are able to change the future by creating it — to paraphrase a famous person who may have said that to predict the future, you have to create it.

Another way to shape our future and the future of our health is to look at the way we communicate and make decisions. Good communication can shape our lives and our health. The way we conduct our lives is partly shaped by the ways we think, communicate, and view ourselves. The ways in which we communicate can have a great impact on how we are understood in all kinds of life situations.

Physicians encounter patients with highly different backgrounds and life experiences that have shaped the way those patients communicate their problems to their doctors. I have been amazed multiple times by the different meanings patients ascribe to words. Disagreeing about word meanings can place barriers to understanding between patient and physician. These barriers can result in obstacles on the path to arriving at the proper diagnosis and therefore the proper treatment of medical problems.

The problem of communication is amplified by cultural or language differences. When speaking with a patient through an interpreter, I often found that a question that should have prompted a "yes" or "no" answer elicited a totally irrelevant answer after ten minutes of discussion. Therefore, both the patient and the physician need to understand the question in order to get a useful answer. Many times when I was an intern in a New York hospital, I would ask a patient, "How much does it hurt?" The answer often was "Too much, Doctor." I had to change the way I asked that question in order to get better results. But I eventually understood that any pain, other than the mild discomfort caused by healthy exercise, is "too much."

This book suggests ways that you, the patient, can enhance communication with your doctor. These suggestions are based on what I learned over forty years in practice (after the end of my postgraduate work) working with patients — and their family members, friends, and interpreters — from a huge variety of backgrounds, languages, and cultures.

There are other ways that you can improve your experience when interacting with doctors in the medical arena and thereby enhance your safety and satisfaction. These include:

- preparing for the visit with your doctor

- taking responsibility for the accuracy of your medications, past history, and problems or complaints

- understanding your medications

- keeping accurate records

- recruiting an advocate

- understanding consent for treatment

- leading a healthy life

- understanding how a doctor approaches diagnostic and therapeutic problems

Recently, when I was discussing this pamphlet with my wonderful cousin, she reminded me of what her mother always told her husband. My aunt would often say to my uncle, "Victor, we have to help the doctor." This is clearly true. Medical care is a team effort. My intention in writing this guide is to help you help yourself by teaching you how to help your doctors.

Choosing A Doctor

Choosing the right doctor based on your needs and personality is very beneficial. In choosing a physician, there are a variety of factors to consider. These include the physician's background (education and credentials, age, experience), his or her personal characteristics (honesty and integrity), and the three A's—affability, availability, and affordability. These characteristics are not my invention, and I do not remember where I read them.

The Three A's

The three A's, as commonly known, are:

Affability — Is the doctor pleasant and caring?

Availability — Is the doctor responsive to your needs? Is the doctor available for appointments and emergencies or to answer questions between visits?

Affordability — This should not be a problem for most people with current insurance and Medicare and Medicaid coverage, as well as possibly the Affordable Care Act (Obamacare). If affordability is a problem, ask about the cost of visits and procedures. Is the doctor willing to care for some indigent patients? (Yes, you can ask.) Being willing to care for the indigent defines the moral character of the physician or the physician's institution.

HONESTY AND INTEGRITY

These qualities are perhaps even more important than the three A's and may be more difficult to evaluate. Quality-monitoring organizations deal with these issues at clinic levels, hospital levels, county society levels, state levels, and occasionally at federal levels. Medical school admission committees consider applicants' nonacademic credentials as well as their academic credentials. I have been told that in some countries, medical school applicants even have to take psychological tests that may address some of these qualities.

Practically speaking, how can you, as a patient, determine whether your doctor has integrity? First, it is important to recognize that some conflict of interest can always occur in any profession. Integrity can be subtly altered. Physicians who work in for-profit medical systems can demonstrate conflict of interest by ordering excessive tests. In contrast, physicians who work in managed-care systems in which the doctor is paid more if he or she spends less can demonstrate conflict of interest by not ordering enough tests. Doctors who are lacking in integrity might also do unnecessary procedures that may even result in complications. For example, a doctor might decide to stretch open a narrowed artery that doesn't really need to be dilated because it is very small or very short.

THE DOCTOR'S EDUCATION AND CREDENTIALS

In the United States, all doctors complete a bachelor's degree and sometimes a postgraduate degree, such as a master's degree or PhD, before graduating from a medical school. The selection process for entry to medical school is usually rigorous enough to weed out the "bad apples" and certainly guarantees that students have a degree of intelligence and motivation to work hard. Most medical schools in the United States are good to excellent. The top students of most medical school classes are of academically superior caliber and probably equivalent throughout the United States. For most patients, it's too much work to decipher their prospective doctor's class ranking, but you can rely on other measures of quality when looking for a physician.

The great majority of physicians take two to four or more years of training after medical school in order to specialize. In general, gone are the days when a doctor could hang up a shingle after only one year of internship following medical school. Now the years of training after medical school are called "residency." So the designation of those years in training are abbreviated as R1 (resident 1), R2 (resident 2), etc. The many years of post–medical school training add a measure of guarantee to the quality that patients can expect from their doctors. Medical school graduates have to apply for these training positions; their grades are evaluated, and they are often screened by an interview and written letters of recommendation from their medical schools.

Further, doctors are certified by:

- the state in which they have a license

- their specialty society

- the hospital at which they have privileges

- their malpractice insurance carrier (in some cases)

- the insurance company that pays your bills in some cases)

- the clinic in which they practice

A great number of qualified people have looked at your doctor's credentials before you walked into their examination room, so take some comfort from that process.

Good training and a high IQ, however, do not always guarantee that a physician is good. Innate good judgment and honesty are probably the most important qualities in any profession. These qualities allow doctors to measure their own competence and knowledge level to handle certain problems. When your health and well-being or life is at stake, integrity and good judgment are the most important qualities in a physician. These qualities are tested during internship and residency training; however, in my experience, bad judgment has never led to the retroactive flunking of a doctor after he or she has graduated from medical school. If examples of bad decisions are discovered by hospital staff, though, they may be dealt with by the hospital's quality assurance committees. Since judgment and ethical issues are difficult to "credential," you should question current or past patients of your prospective physician before committing your well-being to that individual.

THE YOUNG DOCTOR'S EXPERIENCE

When you are choosing a doctor, another important consideration is the amount of experience the physician has. Becoming the patient of a young doctor has benefits. If you can establish rapport with a young physician, it can be the beginning of a long, close, and caring relationship. The advantages of newly trained physicians include energy, their need to please new patients, and their fresh experience with new techniques and recent study to pass certification examinations.

CERTIFICATION EXAMINATIONS

Here, it may be helpful if I describe what certification examinations are like so you can understand why you should have confidence in the knowledge and skills of a doctor who is fresh out of medical school.

When I was in medical school, we took two National Board examinations, in addition to multiple tests in each of our classes for four years before graduating. We took a third National Board examination during our internship. Certifying examinations are also required after specialty and subspecialty training. I had to pass written and oral exams in internal medicine and written examinations in cardiology and interventional cardiology between 1970, when I began private practice, and 1989, when the first examination became available for interventional cardiology. Currently, doctors have to repeat and pass specialty and subspecialty board exams every ten years to remain "credentialed." These requirements apply to young and older doctors. This credentialing process adds a substantial safety factor to the quality of your physician. However, some older doctors have been grandfathered in their boards and do not need to take recertifying exams every ten years. Most of those grandfathered are now probably retired.

My most interesting board examination experience occurred during my oral examination in internal medicine. The examination was structured in such a way that each candidate had one half hour to interview and examine a patient and then put his or her thoughts together and formally present the case to the examiner. A formal presentation is performed with the candidate standing and reciting from memory the chief complaint and the pertinent history of the illness, as well as any important components of past medical history, family history, and review of systems. Next, the candidate describes the positive and negative aspects of the physical examination, the established diagnosis, and possibly the plan for treatment or further tests.

My first patient had some cognitive impairment due to chronic alcohol use. He had multiple problems. He knew that I was being tested, and he did not want to give away too much or make it too easy for me. I had to take forty-five minutes to complete the process before my inquisitor entered the room. This meant that I would have less than one half hour to examine the next patient. The patient was present during my presentation and cross-examination by my inquisitor. That was actually good for me for two reasons. Reason one was that my inquisitor was able to see the patient's mental state, and reason two was that he was able to examine the patient for a finding I had discovered that was not in the patient's record and was very important to the patient's health. I discovered that the patient I had just examined had atrophy (shrinkage or deterioration) of his optic nerve in one eye. This is a condition of multiple causes, including brain tumor and multiple sclerosis.

Because my first examination patient was evasive, I had less time for my second patient. With some trepidation, I walked into this second patient's room and found him curled up in bed and lying on his left side. He had chest deformities, and his arm and leg joints were stiff. It would have been uncomfortable for him to be moved into the classic position for a medical examination with the physician performing the examination from the right side of the bed. He motioned me to come to the left side of the bed and whispered, "They want you to know that my shunt is plugged." He was a great guy and obviously overly cooperative and rooting for me. I did not have time to do a complete examination but did hear his multiple heart murmurs. This time, my inquisitor was a cardiologist whose only interest was a discussion about the origins of the patient's heart murmurs. I did well with that, having just completed my cardiology fellowship a month before.

Some years later, my cardiology board examination lasted a day and a half. One half day was spent interpreting echocardiograms (ultrasound heart examinations), and another day was spent answering questions about the usual cardiology issues, including electrocardiograms, X-rays, angiograms, heart pressure recordings, lab tests, drugs and their use, and case presentations in which I had to make the correct diagnosis.

Even more years later, I took the first offered test for interventional cardiology. Interventional cardiology became another new subspecialty of cardiology. That took one day and was similar to the general cardiology examination but with a heavy emphasis on angiography, angioplasty (various ways of stretching open narrowed arteries), and other forms of intervention. The test had a heavy emphasis on possible complications, such as the potential for radiation burns from excessive X-ray exposure if a procedure lasts too long.

THE MATURE DOCTOR'S EXPERIENCE

Receiving care from mature doctors also has benefits. If well trained, a mature physician has the benefit of experience and continued medical education. All physicians must, and most want to, maintain up-to-date skills in diagnosis and treatment. They maintain these skills via continued medical education (CME).

Before my recent retirement in 2010, I had had forty years of professional relationships with many people and families. Some of my high-school classmates became my long-time patients. Even some people for whom I worked as a teenager decided to entrust their health to my care. Some of these people entered my care when I was "new" and some when I was "mature" but still far from retirement.

CONTINUED MEDICAL EDUCATION (CME)

Physicians are required to have CME in order to maintain state licensing and hospital privileges. CME is offered by hospitals, training institutions, specialty societies, and firms that scan the literature to provide up-to-date information to physicians for a fee. Some of these services require passage of tests before certified credit can be claimed and documented by the doctor.

Medical industry companies also offer training in the use of their products. However, these companies have a financial incentive to potentially skew the information so the doctors are encouraged to use the products for which they get training. Most doctors, however, are able to see this conflict of interest and not be adversely influenced.

Medical specialty boards currently require that physicians be recertified every ten years. As a result, doctors have to undergo intensive study and often complete practice-oriented learning experiences or computerized self-study modules to maintain certification. These courses are often expensive, and if not offered nearby, doctors may need to pay for expensive travel and hotel stays to complete them. Computerized review programs can be expensive as well. I purchased my first laptop computer to study for the cardiology interventional board exam. My total costs to take that exam were probably about five thousand dollars.

Clinics and hospitals may also require that doctors be recertified to maintain clinic or hospital privileges. These kinds of activities ensure that mature doctors maintain their competence.

Getting A Referral To A Doctor

Sometimes instead of choosing a doctor on your own, you are referred to one. Many patients simply accept the referral and don't "shop around" to make sure the doctor is a good fit for them. And in fact, when you are referred to a specialist by your primary-care provider (PCP), it usually results in a good outcome. But you can certainly evaluate doctors you are referred to using the criteria discussed above. In addition, it is helpful to understand the factors that shape your primary-care physician's referrals. They include:

- your primary care provider's relationship with the specialist (e.g., friendship, business partner, etc.)

- the specialist's competence as judged by the referring doctor

- the referring doctor's philosophy of care

Conservative doctors will usually refer patients to conservative specialists. In this context, *conservative* does not mean the same thing as in politics. Conservative physicians will often be more deliberate and not rush into potentially more expensive and possibly riskier modes of diagnosis and treatment as long as it is safe to do so. As an example, a patient may see the PCP (primary-care provider) for atypical chest pain. Atypical chest pain is pain that does not strongly suggest a severe narrowing of a heart artery but may be due to a narrowed artery. Based on all the low-risk characteristics of the patient, a conservative doctor would order a stress test, which is not invasive. In contrast, an aggressive doctor may order an angiogram, which is invasive and which carries a small risk of bleeding, stroke, heart attack, or even death. A stress test carries very little risk under the appropriate circumstances and if totally normal, would very accurately exclude the risk of severe arterial narrowing. If the most dangerous cause of the chest pain has been excluded, the patient could then be reassured or directed to tests for other causes of the complaint.

- *Aggressive* practitioners will usually refer their patients to aggressive specialists. More aggressive doctors will order more tests and procedures than less aggressive ones.

Personality, with an attempt to match the patient's personality to the personality of the specialist

For example, patients with some personalities do better in the office of a more patient or affable physician. It is appropriate to ask the orientation of the doctor to whom you are being referred. You can ask if that doctor is conservative or aggressive in his or her approach to both testing and treatment options.

Talking To Your Doctor

A doctor's job is to make the correct diagnosis in order to prescribe the correct treatment. In order for the doctor to make the correct diagnosis, it is essential for doctor-patient communication to work well despite the many possible obstacles. As my aunt said, "Our job is to help the doctor." Do not leave out symptoms that you fear are trivial. Those symptoms may in fact be very important. Just as there are no dumb questions, there are no trivial or dumb symptoms.

In the modern world, problems with time management, high overhead, and rigid computerized medical records create obstacles to accurate and detailed communication.

Overhead problems, "production incentives," and limited time with patients subtly incentivize some physicians to use tests, rather than verbal communication, to diagnose their patients' disorders. This in turn leads to increases in medical costs and inefficiency in care and sometimes to complications from tests. One cardiologist outside of our community asked me, "Alex, do you still listen to people's hearts?" This physician claimed that he ordered a very expensive echocardiogram instead of doing auscultation (listening to the heart with a stethoscope). I hope he was joking.

Good communication between doctor and patient is important during each of the many steps a physician takes leading to the correct diagnosis and proper treatment. These steps generally involve the following:

- establishment of the correct complaint
  Here, it is important for patients not only to know what is bothering them but also how to make the doctor understand the complaint. An example that I discuss in another section of this book describes a patient who

complained of a rash on her breast. She probably said something about a rash to her primary-care doctor. Probably among several complaints, it was easier for her doctor to forget about a rash than it would have been to forget a complaint that suggested cancer. If the patient had said, "I have a skin problem on my breast that is getting larger and does not heal," it could not have been taken lightly by the doctor who would have examined the lesion and made the immediate diagnosis of breast cancer. Another example would be using the word *discomfort* when the real symptom is pain in the chest. *Pain* is a stronger word than *discomfort*.

- accurate history of the illness and review of systems
  This assures that no other significant illnesses coexist and need attention. Collection of other important data includes the past medical history, family history, list of allergies, and an accurate list of medications (even those not prescribed by a doctor).

- physical examination
  This can be specialty-specific and should be a complete examination at appropriate intervals. There is some controversy about the appropriate interval for a complete examination. Under the new Affordable Care Act ("Obamacare"), patients are entitled to a periodic "wellness or health maintenance" examination to address disease prevention. Preventing diseases is a lot more humane and less expensive than treating diseases, especially chronic ones.

- laboratory examination, if indicated
  Some laboratory examinations can give hints about risks. If a patient's risk of future diseases has been determined, the physician can outline a plan for lifestyle modification or therapy that will reduce the patient's risk of that disease and may even prolong his or her life. An example of this is the lipid profile (the level and the type of your cholesterol) or tests that predict the possibility of diabetes mellitus.

- functional or imaging tests, if indicated
  Imaging tests can include ultrasound, X-rays, computerized tomography, magnetic resonance imaging, nuclear tests of many kinds, or invasive examinations, such as pap smears, colonoscopies, or endoscopies. Functional tests can include pulmonary tests, tests for sleep apnea, exercise stress tests, ambulatory tests of cardiac rhythm, and fasting blood sugar measurements, to name a few. Often imaging tests are combined with functional tests. As an example, a cardiac stress test can be combined with an echocardiogram or nuclear imaging of the heart to give a better predictive value.

YOUR ROLE IN THE DIAGNOSTIC PROCESS

How the patient describes his or her symptoms can help or hinder the process leading to the correct diagnosis. We all use words differently even within the same culture and language. Both the patient and the doctor can ascribe different meaning to the same word, which can lead to mis-understandings. It is therefore very impor-tant for you, as a patient, to communicate with accuracy. Be particularly careful if the "history" you are asked to fill out consists only of check marks in boxes in a com-puter program. The doctor should review the check marks you filled in for the com-puter record. A computer list of symptoms or problems, however, if used properly, can eliminate omission errors (items that might be otherwise forgotten), as long as it really is reviewed by your doctor. A completed checklist can satisfy Medicare or insurance requirements for appropriate billing by the doctor, but this checklist does not guaran-tee that the issues are dealt with by the doc-tor. Your responsibility is to make sure that your complaint is addressed.

The patient should be as accurate as pos-sible in describing his or her complaints and symptoms. You, the patient, should negoti-ate with your doctor about the meaning of the words used in describing your problem. If there is any hint of ambiguity or confu-sion, resolve the misunderstanding.

Here is an example of the confusion that can arise when the doctor and patient do not agree about word meanings. One of my very attentive and dedicated colleagues encountered a patient who became very angry when my colleague said, "Let's talk about your chest pain." This patient wanted to talk about his "funny chest discomfort," which he did not wish to call "pain." If my colleague had not been responsive to the patient's wishes, an important treatment might have been dangerously delayed or not offered. That patient turned out to have severe narrowing of some of his heart arteries and was treated successfully.

This brings to mind the time my wife made the diagnosis of what turned out to be a malignant thyroid tumor in one of her buddies. While having coffee with her good buddy, she noted that her friend had a lump in her neck. She brought this to the woman's attention. Fortunately, my wife's friend took her advice and consulted a doctor. She could have disregarded the advice or waited for it to get better on its own, but she did the right thing and was cured before the cancer could spread. The thyroid doctor asked my wife's friend, "Who diagnosed this for you?" and "Is she a doctor?" My wife's friend answered, "No, but she is married to one." So listen to your friends. Saving a life from thyroid cancer is every bit as important as doing CPR to save someone from a heart attack.

Below are some ideas about communicating with your physicians:

- Have a specific complaint or a *short list of complaints.*

- Define a major problem in your mind.

- Organize your thoughts before the visit. Make and bring your list.

- Don't be circumstantial. Don't give long discussions about irrelevant information. For example: "My pain started at a party at Aunt Eva's home on her birthday..." or "Uncle John and Aunt Jane were visiting from Peru when..." If some circumstances are important, the doctor will question you about them. For instance, angina (chest pain usually due to a narrowed heart artery) is more likely to occur after you have eaten a meal or while you are walking into a cold wind. A heart attack (myocardial infarction) can occur after shoveling snow, etc. One of my dear obese female patients came to see me having lost considerable weight. She was very proud. Had I not asked her how she did this miraculous task, I would have missed an opportunity. I said, "How did you do this?" She clasped her arms around herself, rotated back and forth proudly the way a child might do when complimented, and said, "Nothing." I felt her neck and found an overactive thyroid that had caused her weight loss. We cured her thyroid, and her weight returned. But the consequences of a severely overactive thyroid would have been far worse.

• Tell the doctor about all the drugs and supplements you are taking. The episode with the overactive thyroid patient reminds me of a patient I saw at the VA Hospital in Los Angeles. The patient was a very tall man who came into the hospital with severe weakness to the point that his seven-year-old daughter was able to push him over easily. It turned out that he had been obese and was taking an illegal medication that, among other toxic agents, contained a large dose of thyroid medication. He had lost weight but was also "thyrotoxic" and could have died from this overdose. My team and the patient were lucky that we found out about him taking this illegal medication.

- Describe your symptoms as if you were writing a story. Your reader—in this case, your doctor—would need to know what you are trying to communicate.

- Don't use diagnostic terms, such as *heart attack*, *reflux*, or *migraine*, because the doctor may actually believe you, make the wrong diagnosis, and therefore prescribe the wrong treatment.

- Don't leave out anything that may be important. Many times, an almost "by the way" comment at the end of a long history really pinpoints the most important issue. If the doctor is turned off by a lot of irrelevant information or runs out of time to spend with you, he or she may not pick up on potentially lifesaving information.

- Listen to your wise friends. This brings to mind the experience described above when my wife noted a lump in her friend's neck and alerted her to what turned out to be cancer.

- Make sure that you and the doctor have agreed on a plan that deals with your complaints before you leave the doctor's office.

KNOW WHAT TO TELL THE DOCTOR

Tell the doctor the things that bother you the most and what you expect from the visit. In general, very important symptoms — at least from a cardiologist's point of reference — include:

- *chest pain or discomfort*
  This can be due to a heart trouble (many heart ailments); lung problems; rib and muscle problems; skin conditions, such as shingles; stomach disease; gullet disease; or pain referred from other locations. Angina, or heart pain, due to insufficient blood delivered to the heart muscle will often be described as "pressure," "an elephant standing on my chest," or "a tight band around my chest." Angina may also be experienced as a nondescript sensation the patient can't verbalize, so he or she may describe the sensation with nonverbal gestures, such as holding a clenched fist in front of the chest. (The clenched-fist sign was described by Dr. Sam Levine from the Brigham and Women's Hospital in Boston and is often called the Levine's sign.) Angina can occur at rest or with activity. It can occur from walking

into a cold wind or after shoveling snow. It can also occur because of emotional stress. One of the original physicians to describe this disease (Dr. William Heberden) knew that his enemies could kill him by simply getting him upset. Stress can also be associated with what is now called "stress cardiomyopathy" or "the broken-heart syndrome," also known as the Tokotsobu (named after the shape of a narrow mouth jar used to trap octopuses in Japan because during angiography, the left ventricle of the heart often looks like this jar) syndrome. This is a condition, usually temporary but occasionally fatal, that can mimic a heart attack with both symptoms and electrocardiogram changes. This condition is more common in women than in men.

- *vague symptoms in women that may indicate heart disease*
  Women often have vaguer symptoms of coronary artery disease than

men and will describe their angina or heart attack symptoms in unusual ways. If you are a woman who has vague symptoms that come and go or are constant in the jaw, throat, neck, shoulders, upper back or chest, or upper abdomen, be certain that you have your doctor's full attention.

- *severe back pain above the waist*, especially if it begins suddenly
  This kind of pain can indicate a tear in the aorta, the large artery leading blood from the heart. If this condition is present, it can cause rapid death unless it is treated quickly. According to media reports, several prominent people (Senator Scoop Jackson, Lucille Ball, and Paul Bremer) have expired from this disease.

- *changes in bowel function*, to include blood in the stool, tar-black bowel movements, or vomiting what looks like coffee grounds
  Dark stool can occur because of the use of iron pills or bismuth-containing

substances taken orally. Rapid bleeding into the gastrointestinal system will usually cause diarrhea, which can be black, bloody red, or maroon. Upper gastrointestinal bleeding from the stomach or first part of the small intestine can produce bloody emesis or vomit that looks like coffee grounds.

- *shortness of breath*
  This symptom can be due to heart or lung problems, clots in the lung arteries, heart rhythm disorders, diabetic acidosis, or anemia, to name a few possible causes.

- *fainting or near fainting*
  This can be due to:

  a. dehydration due to sweating, diarrhea, vomiting, bleeding, inadequate fluid intake, excessive urination (as can occur with uncontrolled diabetes), or too many diuretic pills

  b. abnormally low blood pressure due to many causes

c. dangerously slow heart rate

d. inefficient heart rhythm

e. inner ear problems that usually produce vertigo (a sensation that makes one feel as though he or she is spinning)

f. stroke

- *changes in brain function*, including sudden weakness, loss of vision, loss of speech, garbled speech, or confusion, even if temporary

  These symptoms may indicate a stroke that should be treated immediately. Modern therapy can now dissolve clots in blocked arteries before permanent brain damage occurs. Some years ago, while I was performing an angiogram, the patient suddenly developed abnormal speech and weakness. There was a high likelihood that I had dislodged a clot in one of his arteries or that a clot had formed at the tip of the catheter that we were using just below the arteries leading to his brain.

This clot traveled to and blocked a major brain artery. With the help of a wonderful interventional radiologist, we were able to quickly find the clot and dissolve it with a small injection of a clot-dissolving drug. The patient recovered immediately.

- *sleep apnea, which can manifest as snoring, periods of not breathing during sleep, and sleepiness during the day*

  Sleep apnea (not breathing normally during sleep) is a surprisingly common problem that can cause serious damage because the abnormal breathing lowers blood oxygen levels and elevates blood carbon dioxide levels. Most apnea is caused by an obstruction in the air passages, but some apnea is caused by brain problems. Apnea can aggravate several other diseases and can even be associated with sudden death. It often occurs in people who are overweight but is also known to occur in non-obese people. In 1837, it was described by Charles Dickens in *The Posthumous Papers of the Pickwick Club*. His character, Joe, fell asleep periodically during the day because his apnea prevented him from getting a restful night's sleep.

- *periodic fever*, especially if accompanied by severe headache or stiff neck, new persistent cough, coughing up or vomiting blood, or vomiting partially digested blood that looks like coffee grounds

- *other symptoms that concern you*
Symptoms such as a new mole, changes in moles, rashes, or a breast lump (even in a man) should be reported to your doctor. I have known two men who had breast cancer. One was a colleague, and one was a patient who was seeing me for heart disease. Some years ago, I had a patient who complained of a rash that had not been examined by her primary-care doctor. When I was seeing this woman for her blood pressure problem, she

complained of a "rash" around her left breast. When I examined her breast, there was a tumor eroding through her skin. This was advanced breast cancer; obviously, this patient's PCP had not done regular exams, nor had this patient taken preventive steps, such as self-examination for lumps and regular mammograms. I called the PCP and insisted that this patient be seen immediately. As of my retirement three or four years later, this woman was doing very well.

- *unexplained weight loss*
This symptom may be due to multiple causes ranging from diabetes to cancer or intestinal problems as well as infections.

How Doctors Think

Unfortunately, we still do not have a device like the one on the *Star Trek* TV series that Doc could use to diagnose and treat everything just by applying the device to the body of a fully dressed crew member. It helps if the patient understands that doctors must rely primarily on using deductive reasoning (this is how doctors think) and systematically ruling out what a condition is or is not, sometimes in combination with their instincts and knowledge gained through prior experience.

What follows is, of course, my opinion based on my training and long experience about how doctors arrive at a correct diagnosis. The approach is much like a detective's approach to solving a crime or mystery. But in general, most physicians approach a problem in a standard fashion. Some diagnoses are made almost instinctively or based on prior experiences that "blink" you to the correct diagnosis. An example again comes to mind. When rotating through a New York City hospital in 1964 and while on call for the emergency room, I made many trips to the ER during my twenty-four-hour shift. During several of these trips, I heard the most awful swearing from the "holding area." There, the police were holding a patient for transfer to the Bellevue Hospital psychiatric wing. Finally, I decided to see what was going on with this man, who had taught me some new swear words that day. I recognized him as a diabetic whom I had seen before, and I knew him to be a gentle soul. This was winter, and he was dressed in several layers of warm clothing. I reached my hand under his clothes and found him to be drenched in sweat (a classic sign of low blood sugar). I quickly determined that he was profoundly hypoglycemic (very low blood sugar level) and delirious. Giving him some oral and intravenous sugar cured his swearing, may have saved his life, and saved a lot of dollars for NYC, since he was not sent to the Bellevue Hospital psychiatric unit after all.

Besides relying on prior experiences with patients to "blink" their way to diagnoses, doctors can also diagnose some conditions by smell. There are typical odors that characterize typhus, *Pseudomonas* infection, or gastrointestinal bleeding, to name some. Doctors use their senses of touch, sight, hearing, and manipulation (moving joints, as an example) and instrumental aids, such as stethoscopes, to make diagnoses. Recently, when I walked into a room to see a fantastic doctor for a backache, he noted that as I walked, I slightly stumbled with my left foot. I was not aware that I had stumbled. His superb observation helped to make the correct diagnosis of a back disc problem. This was an instantaneous blink-speed assessment based on astute observation, past experience, and attentiveness. Had he been looking at his computer screen, he would have missed this symptom.

Doctors determine most diagnoses, however, by deductive reasoning and the use of the "differential diagnosis" approach. A differential diagnosis is a list of diseases that can cause the same symptom. This method uses inclusion and exclusion based on excluding the unlikely entities. Here, the physician must know a large list of symptoms of every disease or be able to reason based on his or her understanding of body function and how disorders of function can produce symptoms. Any symptom can be caused by multiple diseases, which have to be differentiated from each other. As an example, chest pain can be caused by a totally blocked heart artery, a partially blocked heart artery, tear or rupture of the upper-body aorta, clots in lung arteries, a collapsed lung, pneumonia, broken ribs, cancer in the ribs, pleurisy (inflammation of the lung cavity lining), pericarditis (inflammation of the sack lining the heart), shingles (viral skin nerve infection), or disease of nerves that originate in the neck to name most. Each of these causes has certain characteristics and often physical signs.

By exclusion, the correct diagnosis can usually be reached. After taking a history of the patient's complaints and thinking through the possible diagnoses, the doctor proceeds to the physical examination, laboratory tests, and imaging tests in appropriate sequence. This kind of approach to different types of patients is used in teaching doctors in medical school, on teaching rounds in teaching hospitals, and is published weekly in the *New England Journal of Medicine* (*NEJM*) to teach medical students and practicing doctors as part of their continuing medical education. The *NEJM* cases discuss both common and uncommon diseases. My first memory of reading about this type of thinking goes back to medical school when I read such a case about a man who presented with abdominal pain. He turned out to have a perforated colon due to a swallowed turkey bone. That case is interesting today because those were the days before computerized tomography and before many of the modern diagnostic modalities we use today and take for granted were available.

The Treatment Plan

Once a doctor has reached a diagnosis, the next step is to develop a treatment plan. The general approach your doctor uses should include these elements:

1. *Primum non nocere,* "first, do no harm." Following this principle, the doctor measures the risk of whatever is done based on the potential benefit of what is to be done to help the patient. For example, does the benefit of doing the tests outweigh the risk? All tests and treatments carry some risks. If a test or treatment involves injection of dye, for example, there is a risk of a

contrast or allergic reaction. If the test involves entering into a part of the body (e.g., angiography, colonoscopy, biopsy, etc.), there is a risk of mechanical injury just due to entry into body structures. Some examples of injuries include perforation of the colon during colonoscopy, bleeding from an artery during or after angiography, death from allergic reactions, and injuring or closing an artery during an attempt to stretch open an artery to the heart or other vital body structure. The doctor needs to know these possible complications and needs to discuss the risks with the patient.

2. Decide whether to try to cure the disease, if possible, or help the patient live with the disease and control it, allowing him or her to be as comfortable as possible.

One of my psychiatry professors in medical school said that, in the early 1960s at least, we mostly helped people adjust to their diseases. Today, we can cure more diseases than we could in the 1960s. The treatment of heart disease, for example, has changed dramatically since I graduated from medical school and even more so since 1970.

3. **Keep the patient alive as long as possible.**
A doctor's job is "to allow you to grow older" according to your wishes. Your wishes should be discussed with the doctor. You should have a living will and a directive about end-of-life issues. Decide whether you want to be on life support and under what circumstances if your heart stops.

4. **Practice preventive care.**
This involves trying to prevent *or* slow progression of disease. The best treatment is disease prevention. Good examples include using seat belts, crossing the street carefully, not smoking, having colonoscopies, and not using anything in excess. An example of attempts to slow disease involves use of various methods for lowering cholesterol (in some circles,

this may be controversial). There are many other ways to prevent and slow disease progression. Some of these include exercise, maintaining a low body fat percentage (especially intra-abdominal fat), a healthy diet, not smoking, and not drinking alcohol excessively. Talk to your doctor about preventive care even if he or she does not introduce this topic. Make a plan with your doctor's help. As I stated above, the Affordable Care Act (ACA) will now actually allow doctors to be paid to practice preventive care.

The Importance Of Your
Medication List

Medications are an essential part of many treatment plans. There are many potential benefits of taking medication. Medications lower elevated blood pressure, lower cholesterol, fight inflammation, combat infections, and control blood sugar in diabetics, just to name a few good effects. However, medication errors can lead to serious health problems. Errors in a patient's medication list can cause major complications or even lead to death. Sometimes a doctor may prescribe a medication that is the same or very similar to one that another doctor has prescribed, duplicating or doubling the effect of that medication. This duplication can lead to toxic levels of the medication in the blood. Interactions between medications can also lead to toxic levels of some medications or make others less effective. One of my wonderful patients had a very difficult time controlling his anticoagulant (blood thinner) medication. These problems led to hospitalization and the need for acute care and transfusion. In retrospect, we found out that this patient was taking an over-the-counter medication that probably was not on his medication list and perhaps not prescribed. This over-the-counter drug increased the potency of the anticoagulant he was taking. If he had not been taking this ineffective medication, the whole problem would have been avoided. He could have been advised not to use that particular medication if he had told his doctor what he was taking.

To avoid these types of problems related to overdoses or medication interactions, your medication list must be accurate, and you must understand the instructions for the use of your medications. Your medication list must be reviewed by your doctor at *every visit*. Your physician must also know what medications are prescribed by your other doctors (this is one of the advantages of the computerized medical record if shared by your medical team) and the nonprescribed, over-the-counter medications you are taking. You, the patient, must share responsibility for your medications and the medication list. If you are unable to take responsibility for your medications, someone else needs to do so.

Your doctor and medical assistant cannot possibly know or remember the shapes and colors of all the medications you are taking. Don't expect medical staff to remember "that little red pill" or "that funny-looking yellow capsule." For the greatest measure of safety:

1. Know the names and doses of all your medications.

2. Keep a legible list of your medications and doses with you at all times. In an emergency, this list can be lifesaving,

especially if you are unconscious. This list, if accurate, will also give clues to new practitioners about what may be wrong with you, if you are unable to communicate during an emergency.

3. Bring all your medications with you to *all your appointments* and to the hospital if you have an elective admission or if you go to an emergency room. Having the medications themselves in hand will increase accuracy and safety, especially if there is any question about the medication name or dosage. Sometimes doctors instruct their patients to change the way a medicine is taken without written instruction or written changes on the medication container. This can lead to *big* problems. Ask your provider to change the label if there is a dosage change without a new container issued.

4. Keep a separate list of your nonprescription medications, supplements, and vitamins, and make your doctors

aware of these nonprescription drugs. Nonprescription medications can have serious interactions with your prescription drugs, as we discussed above.

The Patient Advocate

I told my patients that they needed an advocate at their appointments in my office and
that I needed a witness. All my patients
enjoyed that comment. A doctor should
be pleased by the presence of an advocate,
rather than threatened by such a person.
Once a physician patient came to see me
after his prior cardiologist had revealed his
insecurities when the patient's wife accompanied him to an office visit. Upon seeing
the wife, the prior cardiologist had said,
"Uh-oh, am I in trouble?" When that patient
came to see me, he was pleased that I wel-
comed the wife as a member of our team.

I encourage patients to come with a spouse, an adult child, a relative, or a trusted friend. This kind of advocacy provides security and emotional support. The advocate may add important information to the history of the patient's illness by clarifying symptoms and circumstances. A spouse can prevent psychological denial. For example, spouses might say, "You certainly are short of breath after one flight of stairs," or "You do so snore and stop breathing at night, and that wakes me," or "I worry that you may not wake up." These are invaluable historical observations that can lead to a correct diagnosis and a beneficial long-term outcome. A patient advocate can also encourage the patient to carry out the prescribed treatment and lifestyle changes when he or she witnesses the doctor's recommendations. You might want to discuss privacy issues with your advocate and see if the doctor requires a signed consent to speak to your advocate. Many clinics and pharmacies do require such consent.

Change Your Oil

Most of us take good care of our cars by giving them periodic maintenance. We have someone check the brakes, rotate the tires, and change our fluids and our oil. We do those things even when the car is young and new, so that it will run well and stay healthy. How many of us do this kind of preventive maintenance with our bodies? Based on my experience, I would say not many. Often, when a patient had not seen me for risk evaluation and preventive care for an extended period of time, I found that during that period of time the patient had taken perfect care of his or her automobile. Does that make sense?

An individual's risk of many diseases can be significantly reduced by proper maintenance and use of effective medications. Risks of many diseases can be reduced by keeping a healthy body weight, getting regular exercise, eating a healthy diet, and making judicious use of medications.

Your health and longevity are worth the effort and financial expense. For example, you can reduce the risk of a heart attack by about 60 percent by quitting smoking. This approach is actually cost saving because it eliminates the costs of the poison and the care for a preventable illness. The best treatment for any disease is its prevention.

Hospitalization

There are many reasons why you may need hospital care:

- Elective or emergency surgery is needed.

- The illness is too severe for you to be treated at home.

- The problem requires constant monitoring of your vital signs.

- Treatment must be administered rapidly to prevent injury, progression of disease, or death.

- Your ability for self-care is rapidly deteriorating. Reversible causes must be evaluated.

- Rehabilitation is needed for a condition that is too severe for you to be treated as an outpatient.

As with more routine medical care, there are many steps you can take to ensure your safety and the best possible outcome. They include:

1. Ask someone to be your advocate while you are in the hospital.

2. Bring your medication list.

3. Make sure everyone involved in your care works as a team and that communication flows freely.

4. Understand the uses and instructions for any new medications you are prescribed.

THE ADVOCATE

In a hospital setting, the patient needs an advocate, for the same reasons we discussed above, and perhaps even more so than in an outpatient setting. Ideally, the person you ask to be your advocate will be part of your medical team and increase your safety. When you are hospitalized, many members of the hospital staff will be involved in your care. These folks will have different interests, skills, and variable or incomplete information about you. Some information about you may not be in the computerized medical record. A nurse covering for a colleague during meals may not have read your chart in detail. Some important chart entries may not have been made on time and therefore may not be available to a change in staff after a nursing shift. An advocate can help in this setting as exemplified by my nephew who advocated for his mother. He illustrates the usefulness of an engaged advocate. He is the best example of a patient advocate I have known. He looked after his mother's interests when she had a near-fatal illness. He spent many hours at the hospital daily helping the staff remember his mother's problems, allergies, and past reactions, and he monitored her therapy. He felt comfortable contacting her physicians when he was concerned about the care being delivered and the timeliness of care delivery. He did this without formal medical training but with intelligent determination. He clearly contributed to her survival and recovery.

THE MEDICATION LIST WHEN GOING TO THE HOSPITAL

When you are going to the hospital, bring your medications to ensure that the staff knows what you have been taking. Do so even if you have had a preadmission telephone discussion of your outpatient medications. Your advocate should also have a list of your medications and allergies as well as your past medical history. Once your nurse has reviewed the medications you brought, they can be taken home or kept locked up. Unfortunately, you will not be able to use the less expensive medications from your local pharmacy. The hospital staff must be responsible for your treatment, and handing over the care to you or your advocate poses too much risk.

THE HOSPITALIST TEAM

Recently, we have been experiencing a national trend to delegate the care of hospitalized patients to the "hospitalist on duty." A hospitalist is a physician who specializes in the care of patients in the hospital. Such specialists do not have offices outside the hospital bed environment. The hospitalist trend has evolved for several reasons. First, most generalist physicians have found it difficult to keep up their acute-care skills (skills used in treating the very sickest patients). Second, they have found that it is more financially rewarding to spend their time in their outpatient offices, where they can see more patients than they can in the time it takes to see a single very ill hospital patient. Many specialists and subspecialists also use the hospitalist team to manage the internal medicine problems of their patients, while the specialist deals with his or her area of specialization during the stay in the hospital. For example, a cardiologist might ask a hospitalist to manage his or her patient's diabetes and chronic lung disease or renal disease while the cardiologist manages the heart failure or the unstable angina for which the patient is admitted to the hospital.

There are now special training programs for hospitalists. The great majority of these hospitalists are very well trained and diligent, but they do not have a long-term relationship with their patients unless the patients have multiple recurrent admissions to the hospital. When a doctor does not have a long-term relationship with the patient, it can affect the doctor's approach to treatment in terms of commitment. This means that if you are being treated by a hospitalist who does not know you, an advocate can be especially useful. Just as in the emergency room setting, in the hospital, it is helpful for the patient when the hospitalist team keeps in touch with the outpatient primary-care provider. If this can't happen, the advocate assumes the role of keeping the primary-care provider in the loop.

The hospitalist needs to keep in touch with your primary doctor while you are in the hospital. It is also extremely important that the hospitalist arrange appropriate follow-up with your specialist and primary outpatient doctor so that you avoid a lapse in care and readmission to the hospital. This outpatient visit after hospitalization should occur one to two weeks after your discharge from the hospital, or sooner depending on the circumstances. Studies have shown that timely office follow-ups after an acute hospital admission improve outcomes and reduce the cost of care.

Medicare is now reducing payments to hospitals where readmission rates are excessive. These penalties are intended to improve hospital care. The penalties are targeted to save money because readmissions are costly to Medicare. The penalties are also intended to reduce the financial incentive for hospitals to discharge patients too early, before they are adequately stable, after an acute illness.

You or your advocate must take responsibility and make arrangements for proper follow-up. Make this happen. Also, you or your advocate needs to make certain that there are adequate resources at home to care for you. Some people may be better off with a temporary stay in an adult family home or nursing facility before going home. Social workers are available in the hospital to help with these arrangements.

If outpatient physical therapy is planned, be certain that you have a way to get to that therapy. Hospital-based social workers can be of great help in this regard.

DISCHARGE MEDICATIONS WHEN GOING HOME

Discharge medications need to be carefully discussed with you and your family or advocate, if appropriate. Preadmission medications need to be compared to the discharge medications to avoid adverse interactions and accidental doubling of doses.

Doing this is the responsibility of hospital staff, but you or your advocate has to make certain that this happens. Using computerized medical records is supposed to reduce this problem, but in my experience, it has thus far been ineffective or even created more confusion.

I always asked my patients to bring the old pre-hospital medication and the new set of medications to the first post hospital visit in my office, keeping each set of medications in a separate bag or box. This way, appropriate drugs can be combined and those no longer needed can be discarded or saved for possible later use.

Important medications that are new to the patient should be filled in the hospital pharmacy before the patient goes home. Here is a story that illustrates why this is so important:

One of my patients, whom I met right out of the emergency room while I was on call for cardiology, had come to the ER with an acute coronary syndrome. An angiogram showed a severally narrowed heart artery. I placed a stent in that artery. He was sent home over the weekend by one of my covering cardiologists with a prescription for a standard medication to prevent the stent from clotting. The prescription was not filled in the hospital pharmacy, and the patient apparently was not educated by my covering physician or the nursing staff about the importance of this medication. He did not get this prescription filled for about a week, which meant that there was a severe risk of the stent clotting with a potentially very serious outcome, such as a heart attack or even death. Fortunately, this did not happen, but this omission could have been fatal.

So please be your own advocate. Have the hospital fill your new medications before you go home. Do not be afraid to ask questions of staff or doctors.

Access To Medical Care

The doctor's assistant or front desk personnel can function as either a door or a barrier to the doctor and to your care. It is therefore important for you to cultivate a good personal but professional relationship with the doctor's staff so you can have easier access to the doctor and better service. It's to the patient's advantage to foster a good relationship with the doctor's staff.

Currently, in large clinics, it's difficult to have a personal relationship with front office staff when you stand in line in front of a row of receptionists. I encourage you, however, to foster a good relationship with the back office staff, which in most instances would be a medical assistant or the doctors' nurse. This back office staff or your doctor can facilitate referrals to specialists if you need help.

During my first year in private practice, I realized how important the office staff really is to the patient and the doctor. My first office was a small internal medicine practice. There were only two of us doctors after I joined my partner. In addition, one person fulfilled the duties of manager, bookkeeper, and receptionist. The other staff member was a medical assistant.

Getting access to us was very easy. Fannie, the three-in-one staff member, knew every patient by name and had humor and good judgment. One time, a patient called and asked, "Is Dr. Sytman free?"

Fannie answered, "Dr. Sytman is not free, but he is not very expensive." No wonder some patients probably came to our office to see Fannie as much as they came to see the doctors.

Access and personal relationship problems as well as income inequality among the specialties have in recent years led to the development of prepaid-access medical offices. These prepaid or boutique practices ask clients to pay a certain amount of money per year per client to have improved access to care and perhaps specialists. Insurance and fees are collected on top of the prepaid yearly amount. In these clinics, the number of clients is limited, so the doctor is never too busy and has time to spend with his or her clients. In my experience, many good physicians have established these kinds of groups and certain categories of doctors gravitate to these arrangements. The most obvious category consists of doctors who are motivated to have reduced work combined with increased income. A second category, one can imagine, involves doctors who prefer to see a different type of client, such as someone who is perhaps more motivated to foster good health. Other incentives for entering into these arrangements may include being burned out by an excessively stressful, long experience dealing with groups of very ill patients, such as those encountered in intensive care units or very ill people with infectious diseases or renal failure.

Doctors' Styles Of Care

Styles of care vary from doctor to doctor and among geographic regions in the United States. Newspaper articles have examined the variability of medical testing in different regions, and an article in the *New England Journal of Medicine* some time ago discussed different frequencies of use of coronary angiography in Texas and Massachusetts. Why do these differences exist? The same science is available to all regions in the world. Is the science interpreted differently by these physicians because of geography? Why do entire medical communities behave differently when they are so many miles apart? Are patients different in these separate regions? Do strong personalities set standards for whole medical communities? Are doctors' incentives different in different regions?

Possible incentives that may account for differences in care in different communities include:

- There are financial gains from doing more tests and procedures or doing more expensive tests and procedures. This can result in a more aggressive approach by physicians.

- Doctors in one area practice more defensively to avoid lawsuits, which tends to lead to more tests being performed. Some geographic areas may be more prone to malpractice litigation.

- Community standards have an effect. Best practices can be established by consensus in a given community, or they can be dominated by a strong personality.

Once when I discussed community standards with a patient, he reminded me that

Dr. Martin Luther King Jr. and Mahatma Gandhi did not agree with their community standards, and therefore "the community" is not always right. Dr. King and Gandhi did not find it easy to fight their communities even when those communities were wrong, and that may be true in some of our medical communities.

Physicians who challenge their communities would have to present scientific data to change community standards, or they would have to brave it on their own and prove themselves by demonstrating a superior outcome. Even this is not always sufficient to change community standards, as demonstrated by Ignatz Philip Semmelweis, author of *Etiology, Concept, and Prophylaxis of Childbed Fever* (1847). With great personal sacrifice, Dr. Semmelweis tried to convince his era's gynecologists to wash their hands before internally examining pregnant patients. Because these physicians did not wash their hands, they transmitted a bacterium from the pathology laboratory into the bodies of their pregnant patients. Had Dr. Semmelweis succeeded in changing the community standard in that era, he would have saved many lives. (The mortality rate among these pregnant women was 10 to 35 percent.) He was a good observer and used statistics even before the germ theory was discovered. There is far more respect for science today of course, but community standards still vary while the variability rates are diminishing under the influence of specialty societies like the American College of Cardiology and under the influence of Medicare.

How does a patient know whether his or her doctor is practicing too aggressively, too conservatively, or just right? It is difficult to tell for certain. We as a nation need to address this problem. We as physicians must continue to monitor ourselves through quality assurance committees. Insurance companies and Medicare do monitor some of these data, but so far, the local community mechanisms seem to work the best. If you as a patient are uncomfortable with your doctor's style, you can get a second opinion or change doctors.

My patient who challenged the idea of community standards by talking about Martin Luther King Jr. and Gandhi did eventually undergo the procedure I recommended. He had an excellent outcome from that procedure.

Informed Consent

By accepting a prescription, you, the patient, are giving the doctor implied consent to be treated with that medication. Ask about the need for that medication and the possible risks of using it before you leave the office. Currently, some computerized medical records have a built-in system of warnings about side effects and drug interactions. These warnings appear as soon as the doctor types in a prescription. As of three years ago, these warnings were excessive, however, and tended to make doctors disregard the warnings—but it's a start toward improved care. Just as end users helped Microsoft to develop its platform, the medical community is helping the medical record manufacturers to develop their product.

Before a patient undergoes a medical or surgical procedure, however, his or her informed consent must be more formal than with writing a prescription. The benefits of most appropriate procedures far outweigh the potential complications or side effects of the procedures. But all procedures can and do have complications a small percentage of the time. Before you have a procedure, your doctor will therefore tell you about or give you a written list of possible complications and how often they occur. An example would be: one heart attack occurs in every thousand coronary angiograms that are performed, or a heart attack happens in one out of every one hundred stent procedures.

After getting this information, the patient must decide to accept or reject the procedure offered. Usually, the risks of the disease by far outweigh the risks of the procedure that may help or cure the problem. Ideally, an advocate should be present with you during the informed-consent process.

The consent is often worded at a high educational level, although this is improving, so take your time in reading the consent form. Also, remember that the consent is written by attorneys whose intent is to protect the doctor or the hospital as much as it is to inform you, the patient, so read it and ask questions. Ask the physician who is going to perform your procedure or surgery how many times he or she has done this procedure. Make your choice after you hear the answer.

Some procedures are so new that no doctor has done any or many. Sometime about 1980, I performed my first angioplasty (a procedure that stretches a narrowed artery with a balloon to allow improved blood flow). By that time, I was already an experienced angiographer and had attended at least one course about angioplasty. I had also done, with my colleague Dr. Fred Tobis, the first intracoronary infusion of streptokinase (this is an enzyme that can dissolve clots) into a totally blocked right coronary artery performed in the private practice in the Northwest Community. I must admit that I did not tell the patient that her angioplasty was going to be my first angioplasty. But one of the cardiologists on our staff had done five angioplasties, and he was in the room advising me on how to pinpoint and cross the lesion (crossing the narrowed segment of artery with a tiny thin wire placed inside the artery). A surgical team was in the operating room ready to perform emergency bypass surgery if the procedure failed. The angioplasty went very well, however. Later that day, I returned to the hospital to see the patient. When I arrived at her bed, the technician who had assisted me during the angioplasty was holding pressure over the entry site we had used to enter the arterial circulation. In a very audible voice, the technician said, "Doctor Sytman, you really did well with your first case!"

I looked at the patient, and this wonderful woman said to me, "Dr. Sytman, I think you have a future in this field." I was very pleased with her response.

The Doctor As Patient

There is an old saying that the doctor who tries to be his own doctor "is a fool and has a fool for a patient." The doctor-patient should not try to manage his or her illness. This is especially relevant when the patient's judgment may be impaired by his or her illness.

A doctor has a chance to be the perfect patient. He or she should be able to choose the right physician based on skill, education, work ethic, honesty, and personality as well as practice style. The doctor-patient should be able to give a good history of his or her illness, medication, and past medical history and should be able to understand the risks of treatment more than the usual patient. A doctor-patient should know how to ask appropriate questions as well.

I have been honored by many colleagues who have asked me to care for their hearts throughout my career, and none of them, to their credit, have tried to manage their own care. I have followed this advice in my own medical care and have been fortunate to have wonderful experiences.

The Emergency Room Visit

All the elements important for the office visit are equally important for a visit to the ER. Have a goal, organize your thoughts — if you are not too ill — and most important of all, bring all your medications and an advocate with you.

Insist that your ER doctor contact your primary physician while you are still there. This makes the ER doctor not only responsible to you but also to your advocate physician. Your primary doctor can also add important information about your medical history and problems not known by the ER doctor, which can change the focus of your treatment.

When To Ask For A Second Opinion

Most physicians, when asked, will not object to their patients requesting a second opinion. But some doctors will feel threatened by a second opinion request because they have ego problems or fear that they may lose you as a patient.

In general, a second opinion may be useful when:

- The proposed test or treatment seems excessive to you or your advocate.

- The proposed plan seems insufficiently aggressive.

- Your doctor seems to lack confidence or is predicting a poor outcome.

- An experimental or unusual approach is recommended.

- Your doctor suggests a second opinion.

- The treatment used is not helping.

Your Rights As A Patient

You, the patient, are the customer and the boss. You should expect respect, courtesy, proper ethical behavior, informed consent, and access to your records. You should expect that your team will always have your well-being and safety as the primary consideration. You should not be hesitant about asking questions about your diagnoses, medications, blood test results, imaging results, or record entries. Rarely, entries are placed into a patient's medical records in error. This may become more of a problem with the trend toward computerized medical records and "copy and paste" functions being used more commonly.

I had one unfortunate experience with erroneous data entries into a patient's problem list. Fortunately, these entries did not affect the patient's care or insurability. The entries were discovered when I made copies of the records so the patient could take them on a long trip. The patient contacted me about the error, and I promptly corrected the record and apologized.

Using The Internet To Improve Your Medical Care

Here are some ideas on how to use the Internet in medical care.

Although I'm not an expert on the use of the Internet, my impression is that patients need to be wary when seeking medical information online. Patients can be misled, and there is a lot of possibly damaging advertising aimed at potential consumers of medical advice. I suggest going only to reliable sites that have respected institutions standing behind them. Whatever information you obtain from the Internet, please discuss it with your PCP or specialist before acting on the advice or information.

I will give some examples of what I personally consider reliable sources. This list is not all-inclusive, and there certainly are other excellent sites besides those listed or known to me. You should also check into sites supported by your own local, respected medical institutions or see whether they have their own sites for patient or community support.

The sites below have newsletters that can be accessed in digital format by computer or received in print format through the mail. They do require a paid subscription.

- *Harvard Health Publications*: Harvard.edu/newsletter

- *Health Club* from Cleveland Clinic: clevelandclinic.org

- *Mayo Clinic Health Letter*: https://healthletter.mayoclinic.com

- *Tufts Health & Nutrition Letter*: tufts-healthletter.com

I hope that the discussions in this book will be useful and potentially lifesaving for you and your loved ones when seeking medical care.